THE 3-DAY

MINI DETOX

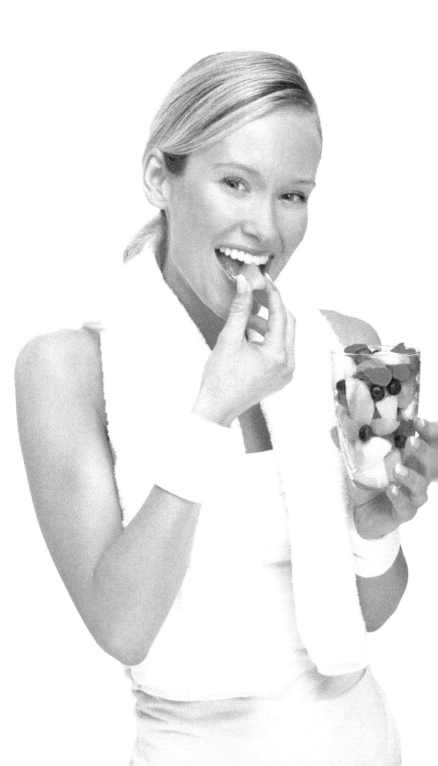

MINI DETOX

THE FAST, EASY WAY TO FEEL FABULOUS AND LOSE WEIGHT

Susanne Grace

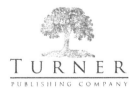

TURNER
PUBLISHING COMPANY

Turner Publishing Company
Nashville, TN
http://www.turnerpublishing.com/

ISBN:9781591203858

Printed in the United States of America

10   9   8   7   6   5   4   3   2   1

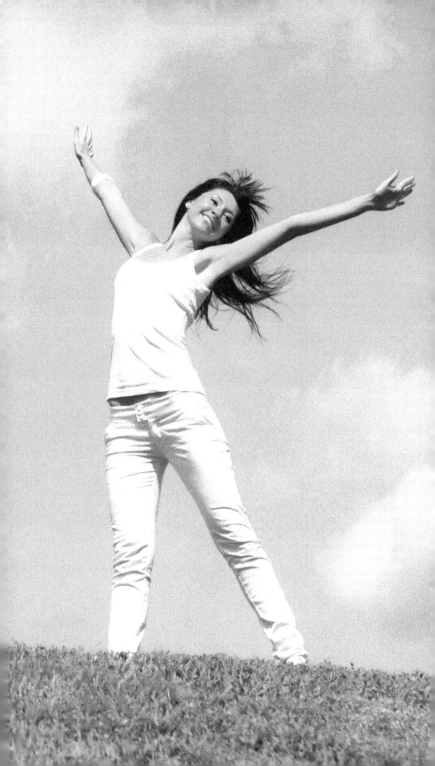

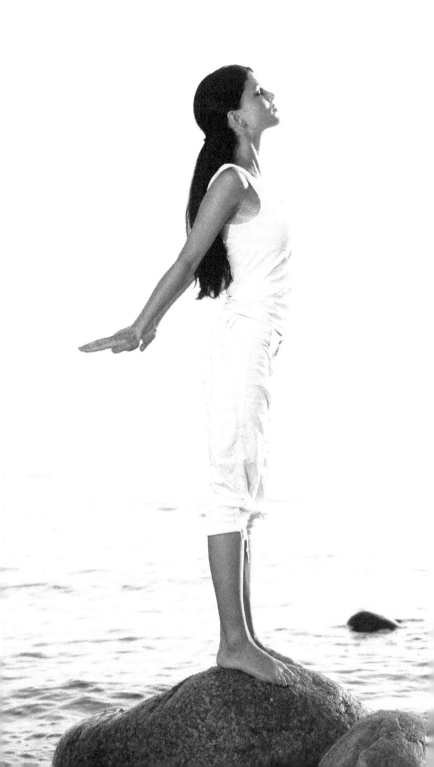

Contents

The secret
to feeling great

Want to feel lighter and full of energy, clear your head and get rid of that bloated feeling? The simple, sensible and natural 3-Day Mini Detox will help you feel truly alive again—and it's easy to do.

Feeling lethargic, tired, overweight, brain-fogged and bloated have become the norm. But "normal" is not always healthy. If you are experiencing any of these symptoms, then it's obvious that your body needs a helping hand.

Unlike other programs, the 3-Day Mini Detox addresses all the channels of elimination—that is, bowel, bladder, lungs and skin—essential for effective results. Follow this unique program and learn the reasons to detox, what to expect, who shouldn't detox and what to do if you are on medications and supplements.

The program's menu is loaded with nutrition from whole, natural foods and superfoods. The fast and easy recipes cater for vegetarians and for non-vegetarians, and are free of gluten, sugar and dairy products. Nor are there any processed formulas, synthetic shakes or packet foods.

The program shows you how to use movement, steams, magnesium baths and clay wraps to help reduce any detox side-effects and leave you feeling relaxed and pampered.

Detoxing has never been more delicious!

Or easier!

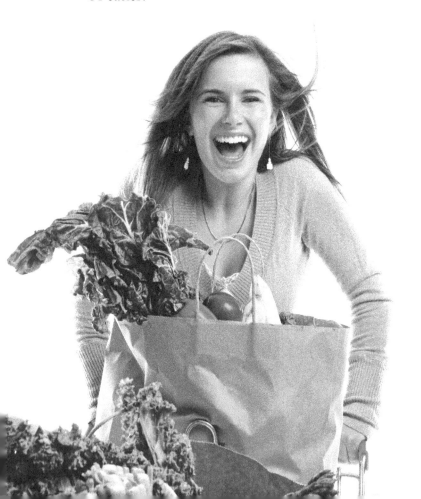

A personal note

Ten years ago, my body was very tired. Ross River fever, almost a year of chronic fatigue, a host of infections, inflammation and pain, and then a hysterectomy gone bad were just about as much as my body could take. After slipping into a drug-induced sleep, I found myself at a crossroads. I could see my body below me in the hospital bed. There was, literally, the vision of a crossroads in front of me. I knew I had a decision to make. Morphine had dulled the pain enough to sleep. In six hours I was due for more surgery.

Yet, despite the morphine, as I hovered above my body, I had never felt more alive in all my life. It was so liberating, so freeing. In that moment I knew I was so much more than that body I had been living in. I also knew that the choice to heal or not was in my hands.

Before I knew it, dark, heavy, painful feelings had returned. Back in my body again, I felt a dampness in the bed. Something had happened. I couldn't stop smiling. I understood that my body was hard at work. The healing had begun. Surgery was cancelled. I didn't know how I was going to heal, but I knew without a doubt that I would.

It was a slow process, a long haul. My nursing training had not given me the skills to deal with a chronic condition with an unknown cause. But it's easy to get sick if your body is struggling to process a constant bombardment of chemicals, preservatives, trans fats, sugars and alcohol. Several years of research revealed that I was toxic with mercury and other heavy metals. I had become sensitive to chemicals and gluten-intolerant. Ten amalgam dental fillings were removed, and almost every detoxification process known to humankind was tried.

Despite the incredible improvement in my health and shedding 66 pounds (30 kilograms), I got sick with liver disease, which doctors confirmed was a result of prescription hormonal drugs.

I had to continue detoxing my body, getting rid of all the toxins that had made me so sick for so long. After searchng the literature and talking to knowledge-able friends, I developed a program that was easy to do and was really effective.

This 3-Day Mini Detox program brings you a taste of what it can feel like if you let nature and its abundant food take their course.

I realized that nature had indeed healed me in so many ways, and continues to do so—and that so many things we are led to believe in the name of our health are only about serving large industries.

Everything we need is in nature. If I had known that

long ago, I would not have experienced nine long years of ill health. However, it all had purpose and meaning.

I want to help you in your own quest of cleansing and healing your body with an unbiased opinion. If you are worried about what to eat and have been searching for safe and suitable natural therapies to help you feel good, then look no further.

Our world is so full of toxins, don't wait until your body has had enough. Cleanse it now and cleanse it often. Given the right environment, your body can perform miracles every day.

I wish you love and peace and great health on your journey.

Susanne Grace

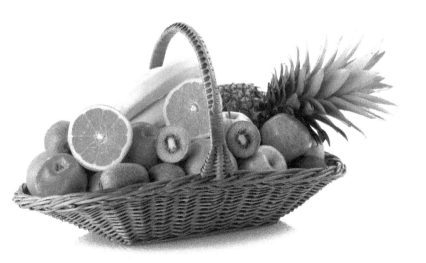

PART 1

The "Healthy" Mini Detox Experience

Most detox programs focus on a bowel cleanse only. But there is so much more to cleansing the body than just the bowel. I take a holistic approach—this program assists the body in cleansing through all channels of elimination.

The program's menu is packed with nutrition and completely free from processed foods and chemicals. Nature really does have everything you need—remember, it's the processed foods that get you into trouble in the first place.

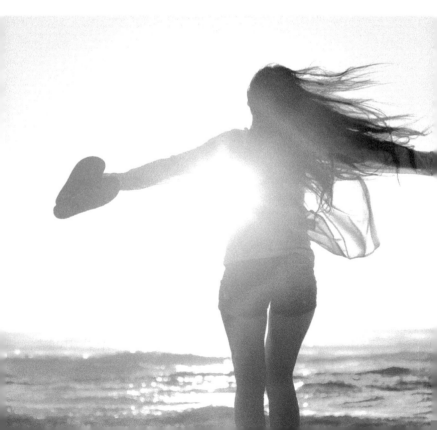

This program is not extreme. It's sensible, nutritious, practical, simple, enjoyable—and most of all it's effective. You don't have to starve yourself or drink powdered chemicals to feel lighter, more energized and really good!

It's easy to follow and by the end of the three days, you are going to be feeling fantastic. So enjoy the process and—don't worry—you won't go hungry.

I recommend you read through the whole program first so you can get a real feel for it and a good understanding of what to do.

Enjoy the whole experience—you will soon be feeling so much better!

To help you relax and enjoy the program, go to this link: www.letgoandlive.com.au/good-morning-meditation for a free Good Morning Meditation. Download it and enjoy listening to it each morning to help get you motivated and feeling fantastic!

Toxins and you

There is no question that we live in a toxic world. Today you are exposed to thousands of chemicals that were not around in your grandparents' days. From the air you breathe, the food you eat and almost all products you come into contact with, there are toxins involved.

Are you familiar with any of the following signs and symptoms? Are they happening to you?

Signs and symptoms of a toxic body

- recurring headaches
- lethargy
- brain fog
- aches and pains
- chronic fatigue
- chemical sensitivity
- bloating
- infertility
- recurring infections

- depression

- mood swings

Toxins in your body

There are two main ways toxins enter and build up in your body:

1. Digestion

Toxins can build up in the digestive system through a bacterial imbalance. So it follows that when you have an inadequate diet, or have been eating foods that your body cannot easily break down—such as refined foods (sugar, yeast, wheat products)—you may start to experience digestive disturbance. This is caused by your body receiving an unhealthy amount of "bad" (non-useful) bacteria.

2. Skin and lungs

Your skin absorbs almost anything it comes into contact with. Once a substance has been absorbed by the skin, it enters the bloodstream. If your skin products and cleaning products are not organic or earth friendly, you are adding to your toxic load with every use.

And when you take a breath, your body receives everything that is contained in the air around you. For instance, you can smell a cigarette smoker a long way off—and that smoke you smell has just come out of his or her lungs. You can't help but breathe it in. You breathe in other people's breath and the pollution all around you every day, even when you can't smell it.

Toxins are all around you

Some of the everyday things that contain toxins:

- additives
- air fresheners
- alcohol
- bathroom products
- baby wipes
- caffeine
- chlorine and fluoride in the water supply
- cigarettes
- cleaning products
- conditioners
- deodorants
- electromagnetic radiation (EMR) from mobile phones, TVs, computers, microwave ovens
- fertilizers and herbicides
- fuel exhaust

- glues and resins

- illicit drugs

- mercury from contaminated fish

- amalgam fillings

- vaccinations

- paints and paint thinners

- plastics

- prescription medications

- preservatives

- processed foods

- shampoos

- skin care

- sunscreen

- washing powders

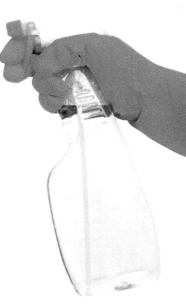

If you're not sure about some of the products you use and you don't know what the ingredients are on the label, then leave them alone. And remember, that anything that goes on your skin goes into your blood. So if the ingredients look like something invented in a chemistry lab, then don't use it. Try to stick to natural ingredients wherever you can.

The problem with toxins

There is an argument that most of these toxins are harmless in low quantities. Maybe they are.

But there are a number of obvious problems about this line of thought.

Problem #1

Each individual toxin may be relatively harmless by itself—in small doses—yet you are getting a fresh dose of toxins, on a daily basis, day after day, week after week, year after year, whether you stay in the "safety" of your own home or not.

Many companies will tell you the chemicals contained in their products are quite safe—and maybe on their own some are.

However, little research has been done to show the accumulated effects of a cocktail of chemicals in your body. Of the thousands of chemicals you are exposed to on a daily basis, to date, only a small percentage have actually been tested in the body. The accumulated effect on humans has not been studied.

It's enough to say that American research studies have found that babies in the United States are born with more than 232 chemicals floating around in their umbilical cord blood.

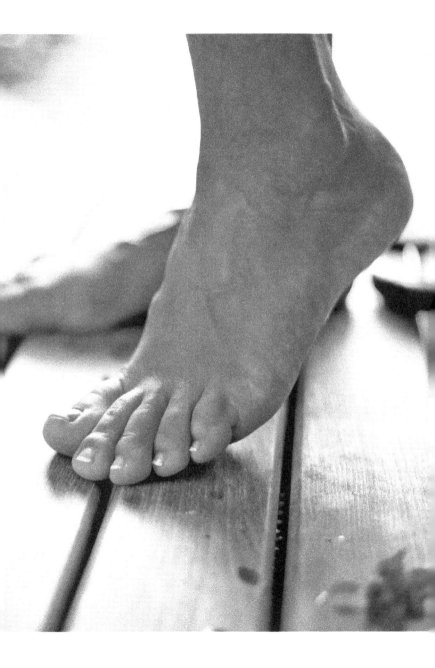

Problem #2

The body does has the ability to filter out and get rid of many toxins on a daily basis. But it can only do so much and some toxins are extremely difficult to shift. If more toxins are going in than are coming out, you have a problem.

Problem #3

When you get sick with diseases such as chronic fatigue, cancer, diabetes and heart disease, or your children are diagnosed with ADHD, asthma, autism and so on, you wonder what caused the condition.

As wonderful as medical professionals are at treating acute illnesses, trauma and emergencies, when it comes to chronic disease—conditions that just go on and on without relief—they tend to focus more on treating the symptoms rather than the cause. And the cure may alleviate one condition but result in another. Pharmaceutical companies spend billions of dollars researching cures. To them that means developing a new drug—and that means more toxins.

Problem #4

It is very difficult to pinpoint which chemical or heavy metal is responsible for your symptoms because there may be multiple toxins present at once. Chronic disease does not happen overnight—often it takes many years to become evident.

A toxin-free world?

Let's face it, it is highly unlikely the world could ever be toxin free. Toxins are found everywhere—even in the oceans and the polar regions. However, you can take control. You do have a choice with your own and your family's health.

The good news is you can reduce toxins in your body dramatically and also do things that help your body to eliminate them easily on a daily basis. Don't sit back and wait for a doctor to tell you that you have a disease and, "we don't know what causes it."

It does not help to deny that toxins exist and are alive in everyone's body. There is no point just keeping your fingers crossed that you're not the next statistic for cancer, obesity, diabetes, chronic fatigue or any of the other diseases that are prevalent in out-of-control numbers.

Prevention, as we all know, is the answer to good health.

Enough is enough

Our bodies can take a fair beating, but there comes a point when enough is enough. We tend to treat our bodies as garbage bins—and garbage bins tend to get filled up if they're not cleaned out regularly. Then all

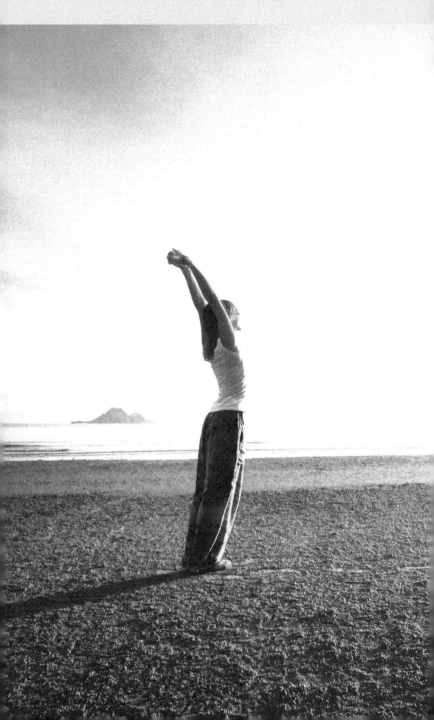

of a sudden the garbage bin can't tolerate any more garbage. The body reacts with allergies, intolerances and numerous chronic diseases.

Toxins are substances that get in the way of the body's normal processes. You can consider them a poisonous substance. Toxins come from the air you breathe, the materials you use, your direct exposure to the environment (like soil and dirt) and from the digestive and metabolic processes of the body.

That means that toxins are able to enter your body from the outside and are also produced from the inside as your body works through its metabolic processes. The level of toxicity of any substance is determined by the amount of "poison" it is likely to create inside your body.

A good, healthy detox is a sensible thing to do if you wish to help your body cope with living in the 21st century—and avoid being part of the population that is chronically sick with everything from heart disease, diabetes, asthma, obesity, stroke, auto-immune diseases and cancer.

Achieving a healthy weight

There's another good reason to detox regularly. In the developed world today, the prevalence of overweight and obese people has reached epidemic proportions.

Many people don't realize that toxins are stored in fat. That might be the reason why it is impossible to shed weight, however hard you try. Many of the medications that you use, the preservatives and pesticides in food and even residuals of cleaning products can be stored in your body's fat cells for a long time after their initial consumption.

If your toxin load is high, your body needs to keep fat to protect you, otherwise the toxins would float around in your blood and you would feel even worse.

So it makes sense to focus on clearing the toxins out, rather than just the fat.

Toxins also slow down your metabolism, leaving you feeling sluggish and fatigued, and making losing weight even harder. And they have a big impact on your immune system, making it easier to get sick as your body struggles to cope with the demands of a daily bombardment of chemical cocktails.

Why diets don't work

Many of you will have experienced being on a 'diet' and been left feeling it was a failure.

There are so many reasons why diets don't work.

The first is that they don't address the toxic build-up that prevents your body metabolizing well and thus losing weight.

The second is that they are lacking good, wholesome nutrients that keep you energized and feeling full.

Take the low-fat diet. When you remove fat from your diet, you miss out on all the nutrients it stores—

nutrients that give your body the vitamins, proteins, carbohydrates and minerals needed for natural energy production.

Following a low-fat diet also deprives you of the nutrients that make you feel full. You then need to reach for another "low-fat" snack to keep you going.

And it's very difficult to stick to a low-fat regime—taking the fat out of your diet removes the flavor. So if a low- or no-fat food tastes good, ingredients such as sweeteners may have been added to put the flavor back in. (Always check the labels!)

You only need to read the labels of diet shakes and bars to see how many of their ingredients appear to have come out of a laboratory rather than a healthy kitchen.

Low-fat foods also put your body into preservation mode. That means it starts to protect and keep the fat it already has because it needs it for living and for all its required processes. This means you end up holding onto the fat and of course all the toxins stored in the fat.

The aim for good health is to take toxins out—not put more back in.

PART 2

The 3-Day Mini Detox Diet

Aims of the program

1. To stop—or at least decrease—toxins entering the body:

    - by increasing natural whole foods that have not been processed;

    - by decreasing foods loaded with chemicals, such as pesticides, preservatives and additives.

2. To assist the body in letting go of toxins:

    - by increasing natural vitamins, minerals and other essential nutrients so that the body's metabolism can do what it's meant to do;

    - by utilizing therapies that are designed to assist the body's channels of elimination—skin, bowel, bladder and lungs.

Activating all channels of elimination

As you eliminate toxins going into your body, your body will take advantage of the opportunity to off-load the toxins it is carrying. When it is constantly being filled with toxins, your body has a hard time getting rid of them all. So, naturally, your body will go to work and begin to release any stored toxins from your fat cells and organs.

If you don't open up the channels of elimination, these toxins are released by the cells but then have nowhere to go other than float around in your blood. When this happens, you can feel terrible. So it's vital you help your body by opening all the doors, and this way you will glide through the detox so much easier.

There are four channels of elimination.

1. Bowel

It's vital to get your bowel working really well. If fecal matter just sits in your bowel, then the toxins within it will be reabsorbed into your bloodstream, causing headaches, aches and pains.

Water and fiber are what the bowel need. So ensure you keep your water intake high and take psyllium husks if you are not moving your bowels at least twice per day (see page 00). The detox program menu is very high in fiber and water so, if you follow the plan, your bowel will love it!

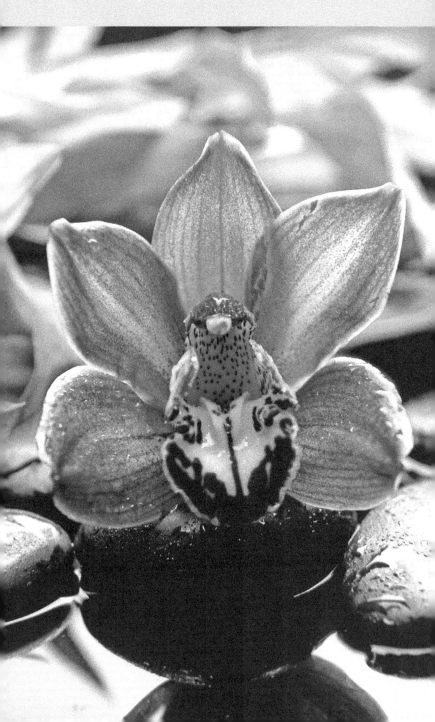

Also consider having a colonic irrigation or a coffee enema during the three days, but this is optional. Walking and other exercise has shown to help the bowel too, so try to do a little each day. The more you move and clear out the bowel, the better you will feel.

2. Bladder

Many toxins will be flushed out in the urine, so you need to keep your water intake high. Drinking at least eight glasses of water per day in addition to the juices specified and any herbal teas you like will greatly enhance your cleanse.

3. Lungs

Every time you breathe out, you are breathing out toxins. So throughout your cleanse, don't be alarmed if your breath gets a bit smelly. It's just showing you that the detox is working well as you are eliminating more toxins than usual. Deep breathing will greatly assist (see Moving gently, page 104).

4. Skin

Your skin is your largest organ and it is often neglected when it comes to eliminating toxins. Make sure you put nothing on your skin during the detox because you don't want to be piling toxins back into it or blocking toxins trying to get out.

There is a good chance that the soap, shampoo and conditioner you are using contain a cocktail of chemicals. The same goes with your toothpaste, bubble bath, body wash, make-up, skin creams, cleansers, hairsprays, perfumes and aftershaves. All of these chemicals add to the bombardment of toxins your body is receiving on a daily basis.

Many products are available in health food stores or online health stores that provide natural alternatives. Try to source natural soaps, such as vegetable or goat's milk. Local markets often stock these homemade products without the chemicals. Cleaning your teeth with salt or bicarbonate of soda is a cheap and safe alternative, and you can always rinse your mouth with a little peppermint oil or mint to get that fresh flavor afterwards.

Leave deodorants alone for three days and let your skin breathe. Yes, you will get smelly! Again, this shows you the level of toxins that are being eliminated. If you want to use a deodorant, make sure it is aluminum free. But the best way to open this channel of elimination is to open up the pores by sweating.

Steam saunas or far-infrared saunas are great for this (see page 99). If you have a sauna or can get access to one, then this will really help your cleanse. Alternatively, a long hot steamy shower can also get you sweating. Please check with your health practitioner first if you have a heart condition or high blood pressure.

What to expect

Each of you will experience this program differently, depending on how toxic your body is. If normally you eat a very healthy diet, then the effects will be minor compared with someone coming off coffee, sugars and trans fats.

I won't lie to you—detoxing isn't always fun. But the process will depend entirely on how toxic your body is as well as your frame of mind. Thinking positive thoughts as you move through the program will help to make it enjoyable.

So let's look at the things you could expect that may not feel so good in the short term—and, remember, it's only for three days.

1. Headaches

If you are used to drinking caffeine, even if only one cup of coffee or one can of cola per day, you may get headaches.

The best way to avoid or reduce headaches is to drink plenty of water, rest as much as you can over the three days and ensure you activate all channels of elimination, including skin, bowel, bladder and lungs. A few drops of lavender oil on the temples and a cool cloth can also do the trick.

2. Hunger

You may think you are feeling hungry if you are used to food high in trans fats, carbs and sugar. However, this is easily solved because on this program you can eat as much fruit as you want in the morning, as much salad as you want in the afternoon, and as much soup as you want in the evenings. So your body won't be hungry as such, but you may feel you are missing your normal foods. Instead of focusing on what you are not eating, focus instead on what you are eating and enjoy every mouthful.

3. Lightheaded

You may feel a little lightheaded if your blood sugar levels are dropping. This is helped by simply eating more of the foods recommended (see Hunger above).

4. Aching or tiredness

It's common to feel a little achy and/or tired as your body is releasing toxins. A great way to alleviate aches is with a magnesium bath. For tiredness, you must rest. Do not plan anything for these three days—forget about the crazy idea of soldiering on! It's that kind of thinking that makes you sick, so make sure you can put your feet up and let your body work its magic.

Having said all that, you may not experience any adverse side effects, but simply feel good all the way through the program. But just in case you do, be prepared and do not worry, knowing your body is hard at work getting you ready to go!

Who shouldn't detox

Children under 12 should first consult with a health practitioner to see if this program is suitable for them. Extra protein, grains and dairy should be included for growing children.

Women who are pregnant or breastfeeding should not detox because it can be dangerous for mum and baby if too many toxins are released into the system too quickly. The Wellness Comes Naturally and Indulge in the Ultimate Health Program (see pages 000–000) are both suitable for women who are pregnant or breastfeeding. Both programs are highly nutritious and

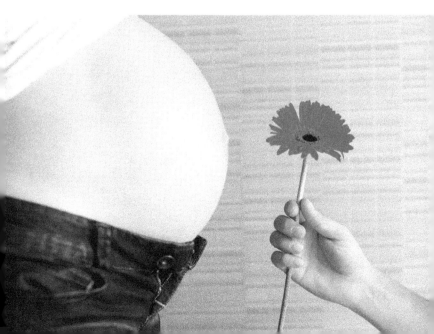

point out what to avoid or include if you are in these categories.

Please consult your health practitioner about ways you can improve your health safely and naturally while carrying and feeding your baby.

Medications and supplements

If you are taking any prescribed medications, check with your doctor before commencing this detox program. Do not stop taking any prescribed medications unless instructed by your doctor.

It is not recommended that you take supplements during the detox. And if you take supplements regularly, it's good to take a little break from them every now and then. If you are unsure, check with your health practitioner before you begin the detox.

The exceptions here are fish oil and psyllium husks. Fermented cod liver oil is an excellent way of getting omegas into your system. If you are vegetarian, then flaxseed oil can be used. So continue taking these oils. And if you don't take a daily fish oil or flaxseed oil supplement, now is a great time to start!

If you suffer from constipation, add 1 to 2 teaspoons of psyllium husks mixed in water once or twice a day— follow that with another big glass of water and increase your overall water intake to 8 to 12 cups per day. Supplements are available at www.letgoandlive.com.au/your-detox-shop.

Here's the good part—your rewards

- You may lose several pounds, depending on how much fluid, fecal matter and fat your body has been carrying.

- ✓ Your skin will love this and can begin to heal and shine.

- ✓ Your energy levels should increase significantly by the end of the cleanse.

- ✓ Any bloating you felt before the program should be greatly reduced or gone.

- ✓ Clarity of mind improves.

- ✓ Overall—you will feel soooo much better!

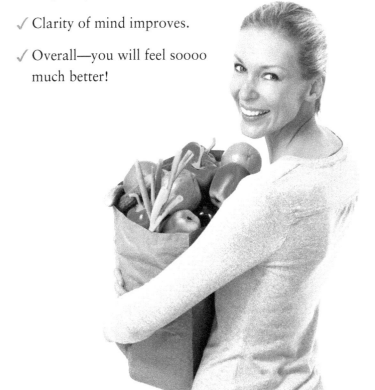

Eating naturally

Foods to detox—naturally

Let food be thy medicine
and medicine be thy food.

—Hippocrates

All the nutrients you need are in whole, natural foods. In the 3-Day Mini Detox program, Nature is allowed to do what she does best.

Packets of processed formulas and bars are not to be found. It is the processed foods, chemicals, pesticides and preservatives that make your body feel sluggish and unwell in the first place. In a good detox program, the last thing you want to put into your body is anything that has been processed or tainted with chemicals and preservatives.

Even if you feel a little lightheaded and crave sugar during the program, you won't be hungry And if you do feel hungry, you can simply eat more—more fruit in the mornings, more salad in the afternoons and more

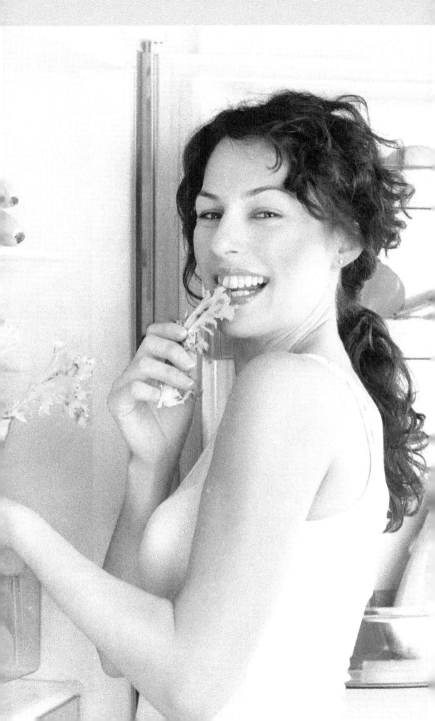

soup in the evenings—if you need to. Sugar cravings should decrease each day.

Fresh vegetable juices are an important part of the detox program. The nutrients in these juices are digested very quickly, giving your digestive system a break to get on with the job of detoxing and cleaning itself out.

You will need a juicer that can juice fruits and vegetables such as apples and carrots. If you don't own a juicer, then try to borrow one for three days—there is always someone around with one shoved at the back of a cupboard. Alternatively, they are relatively cheap to buy and it would be a great investment to make.

As a last resort you can get organic vegetable juices at your health food store. But make sure the juices contain nothing except vegetables—and definitely no sugar. Check the labels carefully. There may be nothing in a supermarket that will fit this criteria—you will probably have to go to a health food store.

If you can't find organic juice with no additives, do the best you can and find the next best thing.

Planning for success

The easiest way to successfully complete the program is to be well prepared. Do not attempt to begin the detox until you have everything set to go. Give yourself a week to prepare.

This checklist will help make it easy for you:

✓ Decide which day you will start and clear your schedule. Preferably you need to have at least the first two days of the program off work, so aim to begin on your days off.

✓ Begin to reduce your intake of sugar, fried foods, cigarettes, caffeine and alcohol. You don't have to go cold turkey, but at least make a start now as you prepare—this will make your overall detox experience more effective.

✓ Check the labels of your skin care products and put them aside if they are not organic or chemical free.

✓ Rent some movies and find a few good books to read.

✓ If you have a bathtub, it's time to dust it off and get it ready for use, or get a footbath (you could use a bucket).

✓ You will need a juicer and a blender—if you don't have these, beg or borrow or make a very worthwhile investment and buy them.

✓ Go shopping (see shopping list, page 88) and make sure you have everything you need for the entire three days. The fresher the fruit and vegetables, the more nutrients they contain—so don't buy them until the day before you begin the detox.

✓ Plan to have early nights and no parties for three days. This will allow your body to do its work easier and you will feel fantastic by the end.

✓ Clean out the kitchen of anything that may tempt you to deviate from the suggested menu. You'll probably find you are feeling so fantastic by the end of the three days that you won't want to go back to eating junk food, so it's best to get rid of it now.

What you won't need in your kitchen

✗ Coffee: here's your chance to give your liver a break!

✗ Black tea: only drink herbal teas during the detox.

✗ Dairy products—including butter, milk, cream, cheese and yogurt.

✗ Margarine: it's not dairy—actually it's not any food really. It should never be allowed back in your kitchen again, so throw it out now! After the detox, butter is better. Don't be fooled by good marketing, stick to natural products.

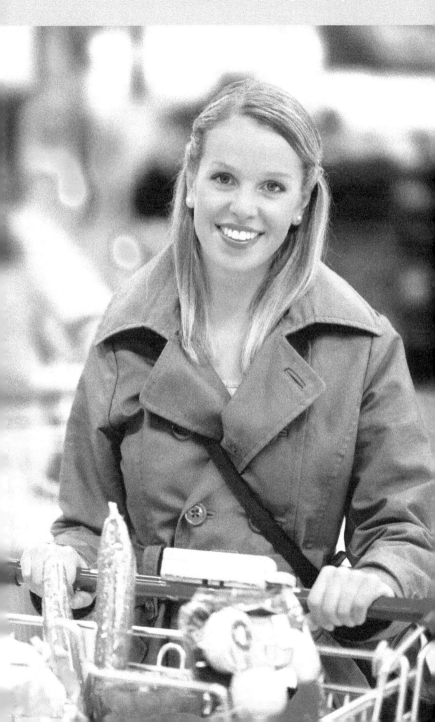

✗ Grains—including breads, biscuits, pasta, rice and cereals.

✗ Processed foods: read the labels—if it's not a whole food, your body doesn't need it. So no packet soups, noodles, gravy or pre-packed meals.

✗ Soft drinks—including any colas, sodas and sparkling mineral water. (It's possible that sparkling mineral water can cause a rise in acid in the body; it can also cause a disruption in digestion. And it's hard to know if any additives are included—you won't find an ingredients list on the bottle. So while detoxing, stick to filtered water.)

✗ Alcohol: it's a detox program, so this goes without saying!

Ready, steady …

I understand you may be very excited and impatient to get started straight away. However, your success will be much easier and rewarding if you take the time first to plan and get everything ready.

It's too easy to deviate from the menu if you get busy and haven't got the right things to hand. So take your time, plan it all out carefully, do the shopping, then sit back and enjoy the process of taking great care of yourself!

The 3-day menu

Here is an overview of each day, with explanations and recipes to follow.

7:00 am	3–4 cups lemon water
8:00 am	Fresh juice
8:30 am	Fresh fruit salad
11.30 am	Fresh juice: carrot, apple, celery and cucumber
12.30 pm	Carrot salad with salmon, sprouts and seeds
3.30 pm	Berry nut smoothie
6:00 pm	Garden vegetable soup

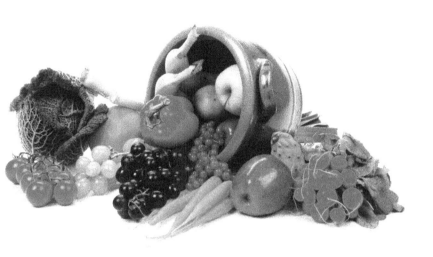

DAY 2	DAY 3
3–4 cups lemon water	3–4 cups lemon water
Fresh juice	Fresh juice
Fresh fruit salad	Fresh fruit salad
Fresh juice: carrot, apple, celery and beets	Fresh juice: carrot, apple, spinach and ginger
Marinated fish with greens, carrots, snow peas, tomato and seeds	Garden salad with fresh herbs, cashews and avocado dressing
Pineapple and baby spinach smoothie	Bean dip with vegetable sticks
Garden vegetable soup	Garden vegetable soup

Diet notes

The night before you start

Cover organic almonds with filtered water and soak overnight.

The night of Day 1

Slice and soak white fish in lemon juice ready for the Day 2 menu. Or soak almonds for the vegetarian option.

Vegetarians

There is a vegetarian option for each meal that contains fish—check the recipes below.

Water

It's very important to drink lots of filtered water during the detox to help flush out all the toxins your body is releasing. This will help reduce the likelihood of headaches. In addition to lemon water (page 60), drink at least another 3 to 4 cups of water during the day. Make it easy: fill up a bottle and keep it with you, sipping as much as you can.

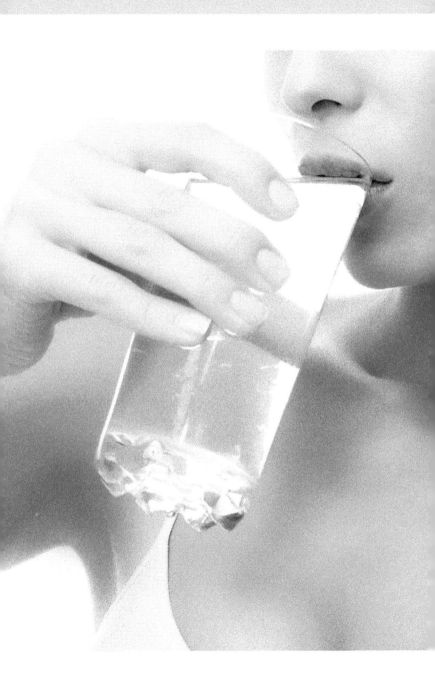

Tea

Herbal teas are quite okay to have during your detox; in fact, there are many herbal teas that can greatly enhance your cleanse—including milk thistle, dandelion, echinacea, red clover and burdock. These particular herbs will help to support your liver as it gets busy processing and moving out all the toxins your body is freeing up.

So drink these as often as you like—2 or 3 cups a day would be great. You can buy the herbs mentioned above at health food stores. Simply blend them together in equal quantities, or just take one or two. If you only choose one, then choose milk thistle (*Silybum marianum*).

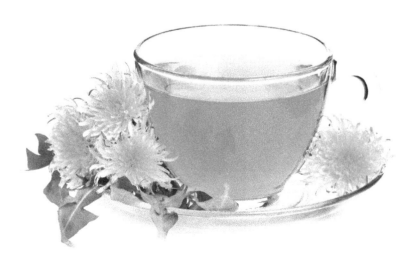

A word about coffee

Many people think that just one or two cups of coffee a day doesn't hurt them. If you have a very healthy body, then maybe it doesn't—for now anyway. But there are many good reasons to stop drinking caffeine.

Caffeine leaches calcium from the bones, leading to a higher risk for osteoporosis; it can contribute to increased blood pressure and disturbed heart rhythms; it can cause "bad" cholesterol levels to rise and gastro-intestinal issues like acid imbalance and reflux; it contributes to fibroids/cysts in the breast tissue, and can impair fertility and therefore reduces the likelihood of conception.

When you go for one day without caffeine and have a headache as a result, here is the evidence of addiction in your body. Caffeine is an addictive stimulant and something your body simply doesn't need to deal with.

Let a highly nutritious menu give you the energy you need, rather than a cup of coffee—your body will love you for it!

The menu explained

Times are approximate, so simply adjust them from whatever time you rise in the morning.

Recipes (see pages 00–00) are for one person, unless otherwise stated.

7:00 am (or on rising)

Lemon water

Pour 3 or 4 glasses of filtered water into a jug and add the juice of one lemon. The water should be at room temperature, with a dash of hot water added to make it slightly lukewarm. Allow to settle for at least half an hour before you have the juice.

If you can't manage to drink 3 or 4 glasses, then just do what you can. The more the better. Each morning you can build the amount up as you get used to drinking more.

Lemon water will help to increase alkalinity in your system and give it a good flush. This could greatly assist with any headaches you have during the detox and your bowel will love you for it!

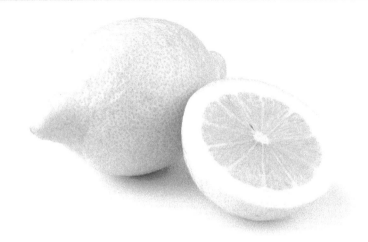

8:00 am

Fresh juice

Make 2 large glasses of juice each morning. Drink one at 8:00 am and keep aside the other glass to have late morning.

If you prefer the taste of different combinations of vegetables than those specified in the recipes (see pages 00, 00 and 00), then experiment and be creative. Just be sure to add in something green—such as celery, cucumber, spinach, lettuce, cabbage, kale or rocket— to each juice.

If you are not used to greens being juiced, just add a little to begin with until you are happy with the taste. Green juices can be a little bitter if you add too much. You can also add lemon or lime; however, avoid orange juice during the detox—and be sure you have vegetables in each juice, and not just fruits.

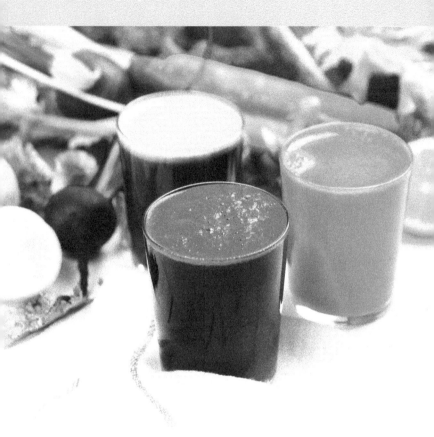

8:30 am

Fresh fruit

Half an hour after your juice, enjoy some fresh fruit salad. Any fruit you like, but preferably no bananas. If you don't want to make a fruit salad, then 2 or 3 whole fruits are good too. You can graze on fruit throughout the morning if you are feeling hungry.

Some suggestions are pineapple, papaya, melons, apples, pears, stone fruit, kiwifruit, cherries and grapes.

Always include berries. Leave out canned fruit and dried foods because of their high sugar content; however, the small amount of raisins in the suggested menu are fine. A wide variety of fresh seasonal fruit is always the best option.

11:30 am

Fresh juice

Enjoy the second glass of juice you made earlier.

12:30 pm

Salads with fish, nuts or beans

An hour after the juice, enjoy a beautiful salad. You can have as much of it as you like. You may like to split it into smaller amounts and graze on it over the afternoon. It is your choice to eat either fish, nuts or beans. Try to stick to the suggested quantity of a palm-size portion of fish or beans or a small handful of nuts.

It is important to soak the almonds overnight to allow the enzymes in the nuts to begin breaking down the protein—this greatly aids digestion and ensures your body can absorb as much of the nutrients as possible.

The salad dressings are an important source of good fats, so be sure to add them. If you don't feel like making the dressings, simply pour a tablespoon of olive oil over your salad.

3:30 pm

Smoothies or snacks

This is the time of the day you will be most at risk of being tempted to eat something off the menu—when your blood sugar may be quite low. These smoothies will fill you up and give you a great sweet treat. They are packed with nutrition. You have an option for a bean dip on Day 3; however, swap this for a smoothie if you like.

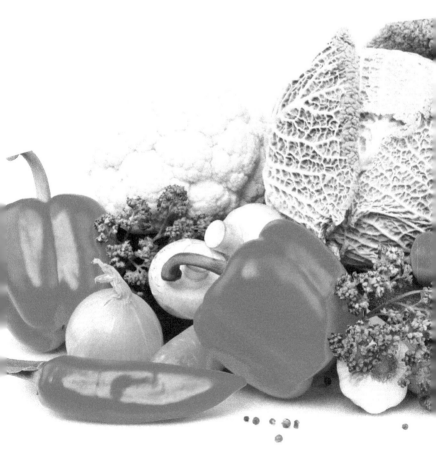

6:00 pm

Vegetable garden soup

If you make this soup (see recipe, page 00) on Day 1, it will give you enough for the three days. You can enjoy as much soup as you like.

If you don't feel like soup again on Day 3, then swap it for a bowl of steamed vegetables—using the same vegetables as in the soup.

Recipes
Day 1

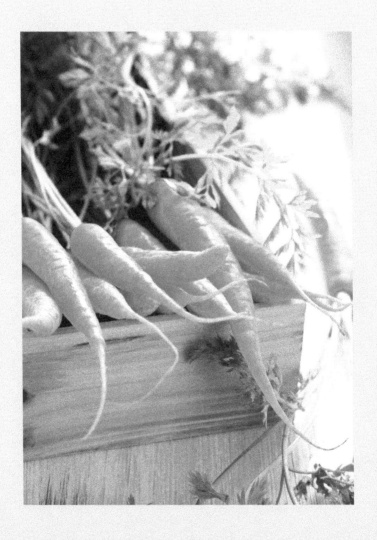

Fresh juice

3 apples

2 carrots

½ long cucumber, trimmed

½ stick celery, cleaned and trimmed

Place all the ingredients in a juicer and process. Stir and divide into two glasses. Cover one glass and put it in the fridge for later.

Makes approximately 2 large cups depending on the size and juiciness of the fruit and vegetables, so adjust quantities accordingly.

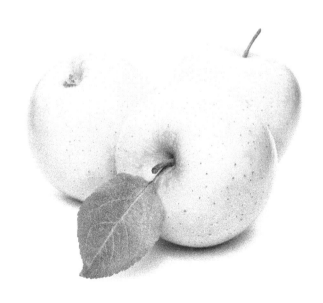

Carrot salad with salmon, sprouts and seeds

   1 carrot, grated

   1 small red onion, thinly sliced

   1 tablespoon raisins

   2 tablespoons fresh coriander/cilantro, chopped

   1 small can salmon, drained

   1½ tablespoons lemon juice

   2 teaspoons olive oil

   1 teaspoon raw honey

   ½ teaspoon ground cumin

   1 teaspoon ginger, grated

   ½ cup sprouts

   1 tablespoon mixed seeds (sunflower, pepita/pumpkin)

Combine the carrot, red onion, raisins, coriander and salmon in a salad bowl.

In a jar, shake the lemon juice, olive oil, honey, cumin and ginger. Pour the dressing over the salad and toss gently. Top with the sprouts and seeds.

Vegetarian option

Replace the salmon with ½ cup canned cannellini beans.

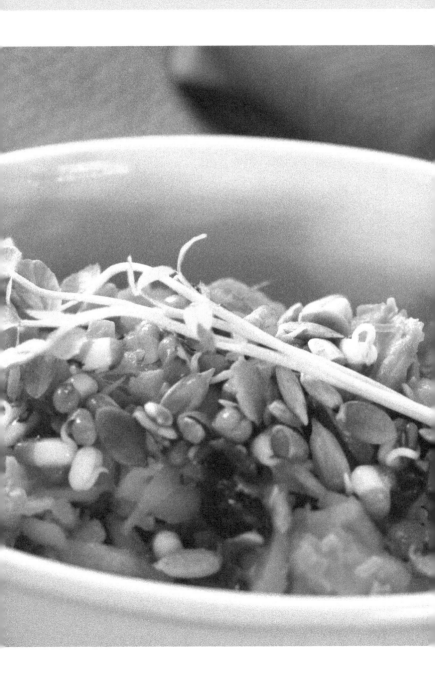

Berry nut smoothie

> 1 cup nut milk (see recipe below)
>
> ½ cup frozen blueberries
>
> 1 teaspoon honey
>
> ½ teaspoon vanilla extract
>
> 2 teaspoons cacao powder
>   (optional)

Combine the nut milk with the other ingredients in a blender. Blend until smooth.

Note: Cacao powder is raw chocolate and is a highly nutritious superfood. It's guilt-free chocolate if you are having chocolate or sugar cravings!

Nut milk

> 1 cup raw, unsalted almonds,
>   soaked overnight
>
> 3 cups filtered water

Rinse almonds well and place in a high-powered blender. Add the water and blend for a few minutes until smooth.

Strain through a fine sieve into a jug.

Keeps for 1 to 2 days refrigerated.

Serves 2

Garden vegetable soup

4 cups water or stock (chicken or vegetable stock)

3 cups cabbage, shredded

3 onions, sliced

3 cloves garlic, minced

6 ripe tomatoes, chopped

1 cup pumpkin/squash, diced

1 cup sweet potato, diced

1 cup green beans, chopped

1 cup cauliflower, chopped

1 cup broccoli, chopped

1 cup mushrooms, chopped

2 carrots, diced

1 stick celery, finely chopped

½ red capsicum/bell pepper, finely chopped

½ cup parsley, chopped

Celtic or Himalayan sea salt and cayenne pepper

Pour the water or stock into a large saucepan and bring to the boil. Add all the vegetables to the pot and cook until soft.

Season with sea salt and cayenne pepper to taste.

Serve as is or blend until smooth for a thicker consistency.

This makes a big pot and is suitable for freezing.

Recipes
Day 2

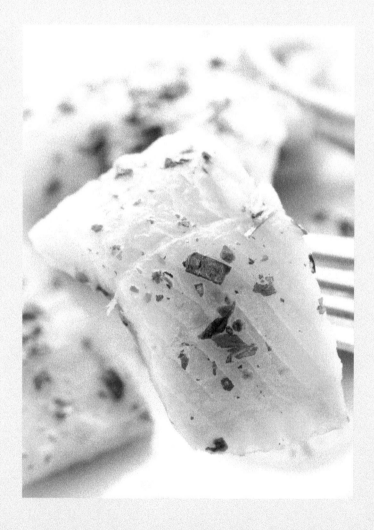

Fresh juice

3 apples

2 carrots

¼ cup fresh beet

½ stick celery

Place all items in the juicer and process. Stir and divide into two glasses. Cover one glass and put it in the fridge for later.

Makes approximately 2 cups depending on the size and juiciness of the fruit and vegetables, so adjust quantities accordingly.

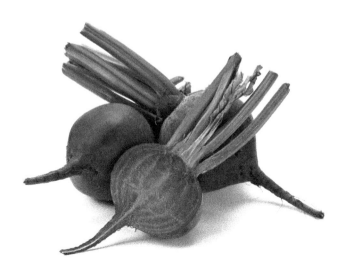

Marinated fish with greens, carrot, snow peas, tomato and seeds

1 fillet white fish (size of your palm),
   sliced into ½-inch wide strips

lemon juice to cover fish

coconut milk to cover fish

Salad

1 cup baby spinach

½ cup snow peas

½ cup tomato, diced

½ cup carrot, grated

1 tablespoon mixed seeds (sunflower,
   pepita/pumpkin)

Place the raw fish in a bowl and cover with lemon juice. Cover and place in the refrigerator for 12 hours (overnight).

First thing in the morning, drain off the lemon juice and add the coconut milk to cover fish. Cover and put back in the fridge for another 5–6 hours.

Serve with the salad.

Vegetarian option

Replace the fish with a small handful of soaked almonds.

Pineapple and baby spinach smoothie

- 1 cup fresh pineapple, cored and chopped
- 2 cups baby spinach
- 1 cup water

Mix all the ingredients in a blender until smooth. If pineapple is not available, use 1 cored apple.

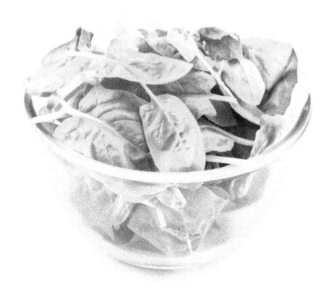

Recipes
Day 3

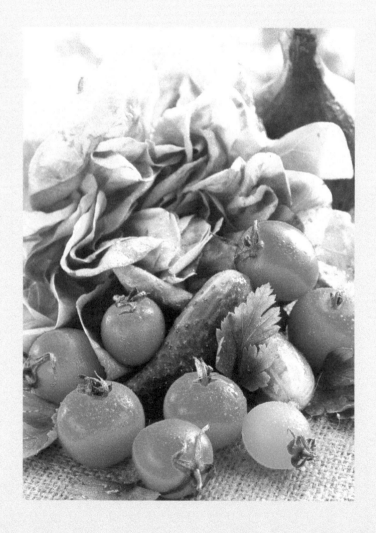

Fresh juice

3 apples

2 carrots

½ cup spinach

1 small knob ginger (thumbnail sized)

Place all items in a juicer and process. Stir and divide into two glasses. Cover one glass and put it in the fridge for later.

Makes approximately 2 cups depending on the size and juiciness of the fruit and vegetables, so adjust quantities accordingly.

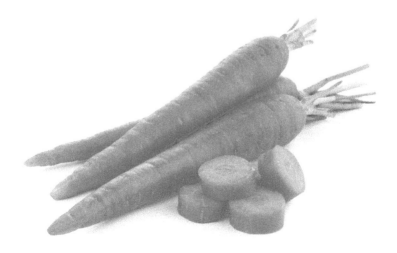

Garden salad with cashews, fresh herbs and avocado dressing

1 cup lettuce, roughly shredded

2 tablespoons fresh herbs (such as coriander/cilantro, parsley)

$1/3$ cup fresh beet, peeled and grated

$1/3$ cup raw, unsalted cashews

1 medium tomato, cut into wedges

¼ cup sprouts

Dressing

¼ avocado

½ clove garlic

2 tablespoons lemon juice

pinch of sea salt

2 tablespoons water

Place the lettuce, herbs, beet, cashews and tomato in a bowl and combine well.

Blend the dressing ingredients together until smooth. Drizzle over the salad and sprinkle the sprouts on top.

Bean dip with vegetable sticks

½ cup canned adzuki or cannellini beans, rinsed and drained

½ scallion/spring onion, finely chopped

½ tomato, finely chopped

2 teaspoons parsley

Celtic or Himalayan sea salt

pinch cayenne

To serve

½ cup carrot sticks

½ cup zucchini/courgette sticks

Blend together all the bean dip ingredients.

Serve in a bowl with the vegetable sticks.

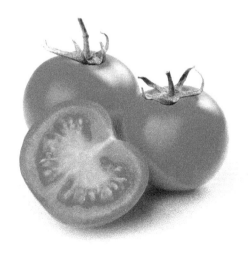

Recipe options

Fruit alternatives

Always eat the fruits that are in season if you can. Here are some suggestions for combining fruits, but for preference use the fruits that are available to you in your area.

Summer fruits

Combine the berries—strawberries, blueberries, raspberries and any other berries that are available in your area.

OR

For a melon delight, mix together watermelon, cantaloupe, and honeydew melon, and put a drizzle of passion fruit over the top.

OR

Stone fruits such as peaches and nectarines tossed with fresh mango are simply delicious.

Autumn fruits

Chopped kiwifruit, grapes and banana mixed together.

OR

Combine finely chopped apple and pear and plums.

OR

Rhubarb and apple.

In a saucepan, gently simmer 2 sticks chopped rhubarb and one peeled and chopped apple in ½ cup water until soft (no sugar). You could add 1 tablespoon sultanas for sweetness if desired.

Winter fruits

Peel and chop mandarin, banana and apple and mix together.

OR

Combine chopped pineapple and papaya (fantastic for digestion).

OR

Peel and chop orange, grapefruit and pear and mix together.

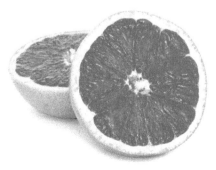

Salad options

Remember, it's best to leave any red meat out of the 3-Day Mini Detox because it is heavier to digest. You can use any white fish or salmon, but avoid tuna, which has a high chance of containing mercury.

If you have trouble getting the ingredients for the salads suggested in the menu, make salads from the ingredients that are in season. And here are some other options. (The ingredients for these additional recipes are not included in the shopping list, so you'll need to adjust it.)

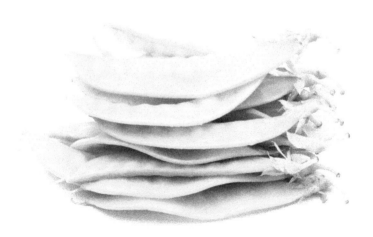

Snow peas and carrots with sesame seeds and salmon

½ small cucumber, finely chopped

1 carrot, julienned

1 cup snow peas, chopped

2 scallions/spring onions, chopped

½ tablespoon sesame seeds

1 small can salmon

½ tablespoon olive oil

1 teaspoon sesame oil

1 tablespoon lemon juice

Celtic or Himalayan sea salt and cayenne pepper
    to taste

Combine all the vegetables in a salad bowl with the sesame seeds and salmon. Mix the olive oil, sesame oil, lemon juice, sea salt and cayenne pepper together for the dressing. Drizzle the dressing over the salad and serve.

Minty prawn, bean and mango salad with zingy dressing and cashews

1 cup prawns, cooked, peeled and deveined

1 cup green beans, finely chopped

1 mango, peeled and chopped

1 scallion/spring onion, finely chopped

½ small cucumber, peeled and chopped

1 tablespoon mint, chopped

2 tablespoons unsalted cashews, crushed

Dressing

¼ cup olive oil

2 tablespoons lime juice

1 teaspoon ginger, grated

1 clove garlic, finely chopped

½ teaspoon honey

Celtic or Himalayan sea salt and
   cayenne pepper to taste

Combine all the dressing ingredients in a jar, shake and place in the fridge to chill.

Combine the prawns, beans, mango, scallions, cucumber and mint in a bowl and mix well.

Divide the salad between two bowls and top with the dressing. Mix the dressing through and serve with the crushed cashews on top. You can refrigerate the salad for an hour or so if you prefer to serve it chilled.

Serves 2

Parsley salad with avocado, sprouts and sunflower seeds

1 cup broccoli

1 cup parsley

1 carrot, grated

½ onion, finely chopped

1 avocado, chopped

½ cup sprouts

¼ cup sunflower seeds

1 tablespoon lemon juice

1 tablespoon olive oil

Cut the broccoli into little bits and finely chop the parsley. Place the broccoli, parsley, carrot, onion, avocado and sprouts in a large salad bowl and combine gently. Sprinkle over the seeds. Drizzle olive oil and lemon juice over the top.

Serves 2

Evening meal options

For maximum effect with your 3-Day Mini Detox it is highly recommended that you have the soup each night. The ingredients can vary according to what vegetables are in season. Try as many combinations as you like and make it colorful—but don't include potato and sweet corn.

If you prefer to eat vegetables rather than the soup, here are some suggestions.

Eating vegetables raw is the ultimate nutrition for your body. So finely chop them, chew well and really enjoy them!

If you prefer to cook them, steam the vegetables—do not fry or boil. Steaming gives you maximum nutrition. If you don't have a steamer, then boiling lightly until just tender is the next best option. Have at least three to four different vegetables.

Spring vegetables

Asian greens, garlic, chard, spinach, asparagus, beans, peas, tomato, watercress, zucchini (courgette) flowers

Summer vegetables

Asparagus, beans, eggplant/aubergine, okra, capsicum/ bell peppers, tomato, squash and zucchini/courgettes

Autumn vegetables

Asian greens, bok choy, brussels sprouts, spinach, sweet potato, mushrooms, turnips, rutabaga, pumpkin/squash

Winter vegetables

Broccoli, cabbage, carrots, cauliflower, celeriac, celery, Jerusalem artichokes, kale, parsnips, turnips, Belgian endive

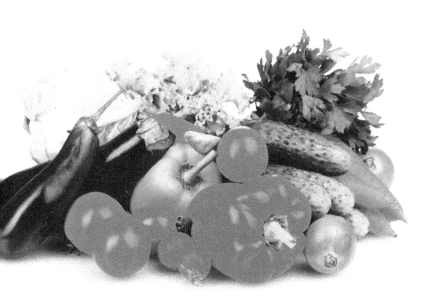

Shopping list

Quantities are based on one person, so before you go shopping check what you already have in your kitchen, consider the number who are going to follow the program and adjust your quantities accordingly. Keep in mind some vegetables and fruits are juicier than others so quantities may vary.

Buying too much may be better than not enough, particularly if you feel hungry and want to eat more. The last thing you want to do is have to go out grocery shopping in the middle of a detox program.

Buy organic or chemical-free products as much as possible and, remember, the fresher the produce the more nutrients it contains.

Fruits

☐ apples, Granny Smith	9
☐ avocados	1
☐ blueberries, frozen	½ cup
☐ lemons	6
☐ pineapple	1
☐ seasonal fruit to make 3 cups fruit salad	

Vegetables

☐ beans, green	1 cup
☐ beet, fresh	2 small
☐ capsicum/bell pepper, red	1
☐ broccoli	1 cup
☐ cabbage	3 cups
☐ carrots	10 medium
☐ cauliflower	1 cup
☐ celery	½ bunch
☐ cucumber, long	1
☐ lettuce	1 cup
☐ mushrooms	1 cup
☐ onions, brown	3
☐ onions, red	½ small
☐ pumpkin/squash	1 cup
☐ scallions/spring onions	1
☐ snow peas	½ cup
☐ spinach, baby	4 cups
☐ sprouts	1 cup
☐ sweet potato	1 cup
☐ tomatoes, medium	9
☐ zucchini /courgette	1

Fresh herbs

☐ coriander/cilantro		1 bunch
☐ garlic		3 cloves
☐ ginger		small knob
☐ parsley		1 bunch

Dried herbs

☐ ground cumin		pinch
☐ herbal teas, your choice		

Fish

☐ fish, white fillet		1

Canned goods

☐ adzuki or cannellini beans		1 can
☐ salmon		1 small can

Nuts and seeds

☐ almonds, raw unsalted		1 cup
☐ cashews, raw unsalted		½ cup
☐ pepita/pumpkin seeds		2 Tbs
☐ sunflower seeds		2 Tbs

Fats

☐ olive oil	½ cup

Condiments

☐ cacao powder	2 tsp
☐ cayenne pepper	to taste
☐ sea salt	to taste
☐ coconut milk	1 small can
☐ raisins	1 Tbs
☐ raw natural honey	2 tsp
☐ vanilla extract	½ tsp
☐ vegetable or chicken stock (preferably homemade or organic powdered)	4 cups

Vegetarian options

☐ extra almonds	½ cup
☐ cannellini beans, canned	½ cup

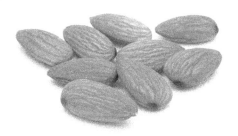

PART 3

Enhancing the Detox

Day spa therapies

To help make this the ultimate 3-Day Mini Detox, the highly nutritious menu is very effective, but you can do even better.

Your whole body deserves some time out as well as some nurturing while you are moving through the cleansing process.

The following therapies are simply to help you make the most out of the detox experience. It's up to you whether you use them and how often. As a minimum though, I recommend magnesium baths or footbaths as well as a clay wrap.

Magnesium baths or footbaths

Each day on your detox program have either a magnesium chloride or a magnesium sulfate (better know as Epsom salts) bath.

Epsom salts are wonderful for helping to relieve aches and pains and draw out toxins. But magnesium chloride is the Rolls-Royce of magnesium—it's highly absorbable, giving your body a great dose of magnesium in the process.

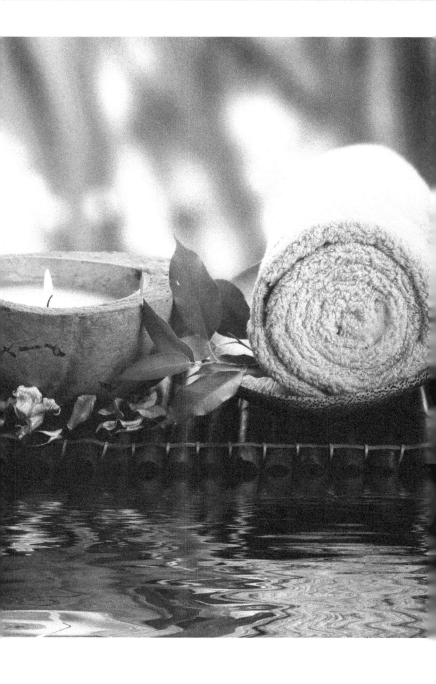

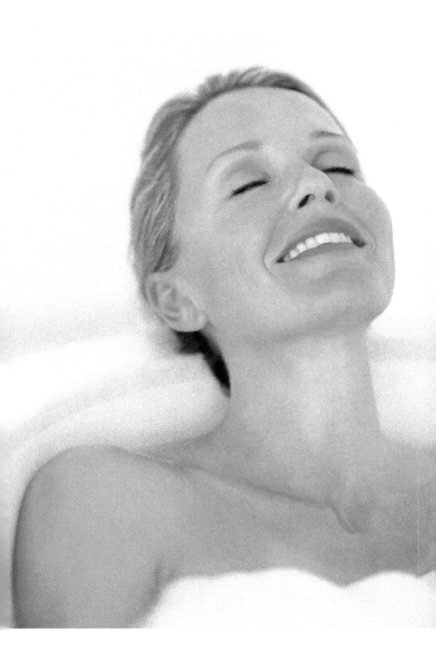

The benefits of magnesium go beyond feeling calm, relaxed and the relief of aching muscles and joints. Magnesium is essential for over 300 functions in your body.

Inadequate intake of magnesium has been linked to various adverse health outcomes, including cardio-vascular disease, hypertension, diabetes mellitus and headaches. Magnesium is also important in bone growth and may play a role in athletic performance.

If you don't have a bathtub, get a bucket and have a footbath. Use 1 to 2 cups of magnesium in a bath and ½ cup in a footbath. Soak your feet for 20 to 30 minutes.

Light some of your favorite candles and play sooth-ing music to make the whole experience more relaxing and delightful.

Warning

Please make sure you avoid hot mineral baths if you have circulation or blood pressure problems. Strong heat and salt should also be avoided in pregnancy.

Clay wrap

Bentonite clay is the ultimate in clays. It acts like a mag-net—drawing out heavy metals, chemicals and toxins through your skin. You can put the clay in your bath or footbath in the same quantities as the magnesium.

Or mix the clay and the magnesium together for the ultimate detox bath.

Alternatively, mix the clay with a little filtered water into a thick yogurt-like consistency and rub it all over your body, focusing first on the chest and back and particularly under the arms and groin where your lymph glands are. Then lie down on an old sheet on top of a yoga mat and wrap yourself up. Lie there for up to an hour and relax as the clay gets to work and pulls toxins out through your skin.

In the last 15 minutes, apply some of the left-over mixed clay to your face—it's a fabulous face mask and draws out all impurities. Simply shower the clay off, using no soap, only water.

If your skin feels a little dry, apply a small amount of coconut oil—it's good enough to eat!

This is a fantastic therapy to use with the detox. I recommend you do this on Day 2.

Saunas

Wet steam saunas are an effective way of cleansing the body. In fact if you could choose only one therapy, it would be this one. Unfortunately, not everyone has a sauna in their own home or has access to one. But if you do, then please use it daily while on your detox program. It will greatly increase the toxins that are moving out from every pore in your skin as you sweat it out.

Wet steams are generally more comfortable than dry saunas, and the ultimate would have to be the far-infrared sauna.

Infrared energy helps your skin to release toxins through a process called "resonant absorption." This means that the frequency of the far-infrared energy matches the frequency of the water in your cells. This then draws out the toxins into the bloodstream to be released in your sweat.

Make sure with any sauna that you take a dose of either colloidal minerals or half a cup of salty water (using sea salt). This will replace any minerals you lose through sweating.

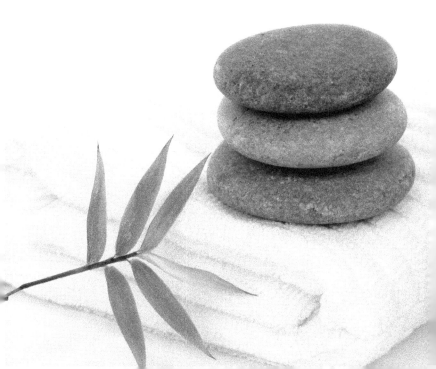

Other therapies to consider

Dry skin brushing

Dry skin brushing carries toxins to where they can be eliminated by the kidneys, liver and bowels, as well as through the skin. It's good for anyone who wants to improve their general wellbeing. It's especially beneficial for people who have a sluggish system or who are not very physically active.

The best time to skin-brush is before you take a shower or bath. Do this daily for 2 to 5 minutes until your skin is rosy pink using a natural fiber-skin brush. Avoid brushing areas where there is inflamed, broken or irritated skin.

Always brush towards the heart because your lymph system moves fluid in this direction—this means you need to use "upward" brushstrokes. The common pathway for brushing is from your feet to your nipple region, from your hands towards your shoulders and from your face towards your chest. Use long strokes where you can, and finish the strokes near a lymph node.

Colonic irrigations

Colonic irrigation is administered by a qualified professional to irrigate and cleanse your colon with water. The water is warmed and gentle pressure is used to remove toxins and waste products from your colon.

When you've had a sluggish digestive system and highly refined diet, your bowel stores waste particles and toxins that often end up back in your bloodstream. This therapy gives your colon an overhaul and a chance to start fresh with your new way of living.

Having a colonic irrigation in conjunction with the 3-Day Mini Detox can greatly enhance the detoxifying process and reduce cleansing symptoms such as headaches, aches and pains.

Coffee enemas

Coffee enemas are beneficial in reducing the toxic load your liver is trying to deal with, as well as cleansing the whole body. They can be particularly effective when they are used in conjunction with a cleansing program.

Massage

Massage not only feels nice, it's good for you too. Massage increases circulation of your blood and lymph. This means it takes blood where it needs to go and helps to remove toxins. Massage works on your nervous system to help it relax and it helps your muscles and tendons to let go of stress.

When you have better circulation, a larger quantity of oxygen and nutrients is being carried around to your muscles and organs. This increases your body's ability to release stress and toxins and for your organs to receive all the nutrients they need to function properly.

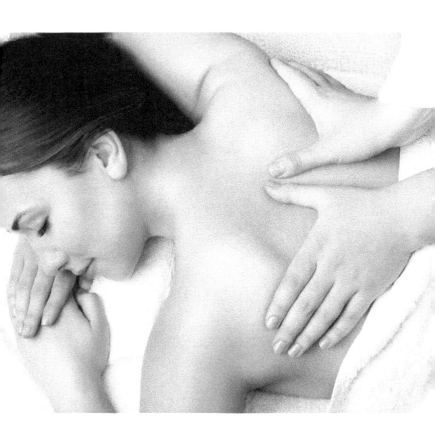

There are so many wonderful day spa therapies you can do at home easily and cheaply. They form part of our larger programs: Wellness Comes Naturally (49 days) and Indulge in the Ultimate Health Program. Therapies such as skin scrubs, seaweed baths, hydrotherapy, hair and skin care, aromatherapy, energy healing and poultices are incorporated into these programs' home spa menus and are demonstrated on video (see pages 000–000).

Moving and thinking

Moving gently

No marathons are needed. In fact, if you are an active person, then these three days should be taken as a rest. Gentle stretching, walking and breathing will be the most effective way to assist your body as it releases toxins during the detox. Take it nice and slow. Gentle movement is what you want to aim for—doing a gym workout will not help your body right now.

1. Stretching

Not only during your mini detox but at all times, it is great to begin your day with some stretches to help wake up your body. So take the time and slowly and gently stretch all the major muscles in your body.

Move your arms around, and gently stretch your neck, your spine, hips and legs. Just do what feels natural and easy, in your own time. Even ten minutes of stretching will leave you feeling better.

2. Walking

Walking is a great way to get your body moving and the circulation going. If you can manage it, first thing in

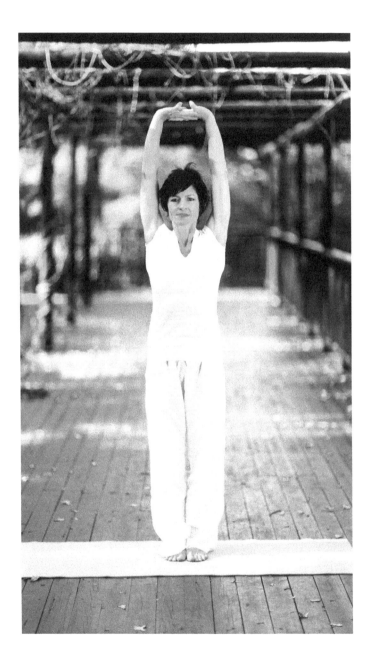

the morning is a great time for walking, otherwise any time throughout the day—just try and get in at least a 15-minute walk. This will move your lymph and blood and really help your body to move those toxins out.

3. Deep breathing

Doing some deep breathing as you walk really helps to eliminate toxins through your breath. Alternatively, you can sit down and slowly deep-breathe whenever you think of it through the day.

Remember, your lungs are one way your body eliminates toxins and—since you are releasing many toxins during the program, you may as well help your body along and breathe deeply!

Being grateful

There is so much to be grateful for. Take just 5 minutes each morning as you drink your lemon water and stop to give thanks to your body. You may have been neglecting it, you may have been giving it a battering. It's time now to give it thanks instead. It's been doing the best it can do, regardless of what you do to it, so nurture your body and give it a hug!

Don't forget, you have the Good Morning Meditation to listen to each morning—this will really help to get you into a great space and it only takes 10 minutes. (See page 00 for the link.)

Bringing it all together

Here is a simple chart bringing all the elements together. Simply tick it off as you go to be sure you get the most out of the program.

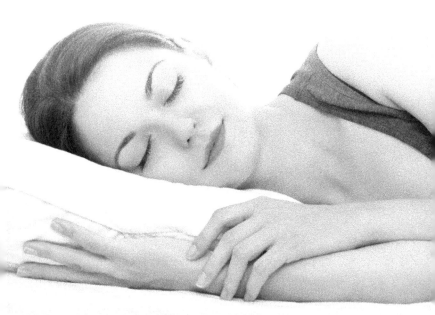

Days	1	2	3
10-minute stretch			
Lemon water			
5-minute contemplation			
Juice			
Fruit			
Juice			
Salad			
Smoothie/snack			
Soup			
Walking			
Deep breathing			
Bath or footbath (daily)			
Clay wrap (1 day only)			
Sauna if available (daily)			
Food preparation for tomorrow			
Early to bed!			

PART 4

Staying Healthy,
Learning More

During the 3-Day Mini Detox program I hope you have got a lot of new ideas and information and will find ways to incorporate them into your daily life.

You may not want to go straight back to how you were eating before. Slowly add in healthy grains and more proteins, good fats and healthy dairy.

Continue having a green juice and/or smoothie every day, and aim to have at least 50 percent of your meals raw—fresh fruit, salads, nuts and seeds. Your body will love you for it! Enjoy the abundance of foods that nature has to offer, be curious about recipes, experiment and have fun.

You are often told that certain foods are good for you, when in fact they are highly processed or nutrient poor. Eating low-fat foods, or replacing butter with margarine are just two examples of unhealthy diet trends fueled by misinformation. These trends can lead you to becoming fat and toxic, and eventually reaching for quick fixes and embarking on yo-yo diets.

Here are some simple ways you can swap unhealthy food for healthy food.

Swap this	For that
Margarine/processed spreads	Butter
Table salt	Celtic sea salt or Himalayan salt
Canola oil/vegetable oils	Coconut oil/extra virgin olive oil
Low-fat dairy	Full-cream dairy
Processed cheese	Fermented cheese (e.g., brie, camembert, feta)
Processed and packaged foods	Whole foods (unprocessed)
Non-organic produce	Organic produce where possible
Processed soy products	Naturally fermented soy products
Wheat: white breads	Whole grains: spelt, barley, rye, sourdough bread

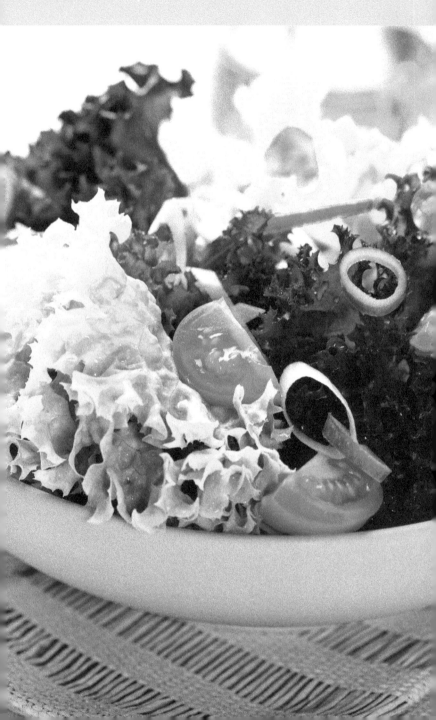

Want to learn more?

Recommended reading

Adal A. "Heavy Metal Toxicity." *Medscape,* Jan 2014; see http://emedicine.medscape.com/article/814960-overview.

Baker N. *The Body Toxic: How the Hazardous Chemistry of Everyday Things Threatens Our Health and Wellbeing.* New York: North Point Press, 2009.

Bijlsma N. *Healthy Home Healthy Family: Is Where You Live Affecting Your Health?* Buddina, Queensland, AU: Joshua Books, 2010.

Crinnion W. *Clean, Green & Lean.* New York: John Wiley & Sons Inc., 2010.

Davis E. "Health Hazards of Mercury." *Wise Traditions.* Weston A. Price Foundation, Dec 8, 2003; see www.westonaprice.org/environmental-toxins/health-hazards-of-mercury.

Fallon S. *Nourishing Traditions: The Cookbook That Challenges Politically Correct Nutrition and the Diet Dictocrats.* 2nd ed. Washington, DC: New Trends Publishing, 2003.

Frazer D. *Firstly, Do No Harm: A Classic Adventure into Health and Healing.* Engadine, NSW, AU: Dale Frazer Publisher, 1999.

Ginsberg G, B Toal. *What's Toxic, What's Not.* New York: Berkley Trade, 2006.

Health and Environment Alliance. "Mercury and Vaccines." Fact Sheet, Oct 2006; see www.env-health.org/IMG/pdf/Mercury_and_vaccines.pdf.

Houston MC. "Role of Mercury Toxicity in Hypertension, Cardiovascular Disease, and Stroke." Abstract. *National Center for Biotechnology Information,* Aug 2011; see www.ncbi.nlm.nih.gov/pubmed/21806773.

Koral SM. "The Scientific Case Against Amalgam." International Academy of Oral Medicine & Toxicology, 2002/2005; see www.fda.gov/ohrms/dockets/dockets/06n0352/06N-0352-EC22-Attach-28.pdf.

Krohn J, F Taylor. *Natural Detoxification: A Practical Encyclopedia.* Columbus, OH: The Educational Publisher/Biblio Publishing, 2013.

Lantz S. *Chemical Free Kids: Raising Healthy Children in a Toxic World.* Buddina, Queensland, AU: Joshua Books, 2009.

Lourie B, R Smith. *Slow Death by Rubber Duck: The Secret Danger of Everyday Things.* Berkeley, CA: Counterpoint, 2009.

"Mercury Dental Amalgams Banned in 3 Countries: FDA, EPA, ADA Still Allow and Encourage Heavy-Metal Fillings." *Orthomolecular Medicine News Service,* Nov 2008; see http://orthomolecular.org/resources/omns/v04n24.shtml.

"Mercury in the Household." Ohio Environmental Protection Agency, Jun 2010; see http://medinahealth.org/images/company_assets/d98a6e31-3e37-43ff-bc1a-ecc84e8f1117/OEPAMercuryinHousehold2010_dc57.PDF.

O'Brien J. "Mercury Amalgam Toxicity." International Center for Nutritional Research; see www.icnr.com/articles/mercuryamalgamtoxicity.html.

Rull G. "Heavy Metal Poisoning." *Patient.co.uk,* May 2009; see www.patient.co.uk/doctor/heavy-metal-poisoning.

Schmid R. *Traditional Foods Are Your Best Medicine.* Rochester, VT: Healing Arts Press, 1997.

My notes and dreams

As you detox your body on a physical level, don't be surprised if some emotions rise up for you too. Your physical cells are where you store buried emotions that you have not been able to express. You can tell your physical body is linked to emotions just by the fact that you can get "butterflies" in the tummy, or even feel sick when you are nervous.

So throughout your 3-Day Mini Detox, to help you detox on all levels, use the following pages to write out any feelings that may arise. Just notice how you are feeling and be aware that feeling cranky or frustrated is part of the detox journey—and it's all good!

It's better to let these feelings out, so rather than take them out on those around you, write them down and let them go. You'll feel soooo much better!

Advanced detox programs

Three days is a great start, but there's so much more to explore! If you would like a stack more incredibly healthy easy recipes, suggested menus, day spa menus, and step-by-step instructions to really enhance your health and have you feeling absolutely fabulous, then you have the choice of several programs.

Go to www.letgoandlive.com.au and explore the many benefits my programs can give you.

The 10-Day Spring Clean

If you would like to feel even lighter and drop a dress size or two, then you can in only 10 days (with the option to do only seven days). You will feel lighter, your skin will be clearer, your mind clear and you'll be full of energy.

This program features a delicious raw food menu that is cleansing for your body. You will learn more day spa therapies that you can do at home, you get a

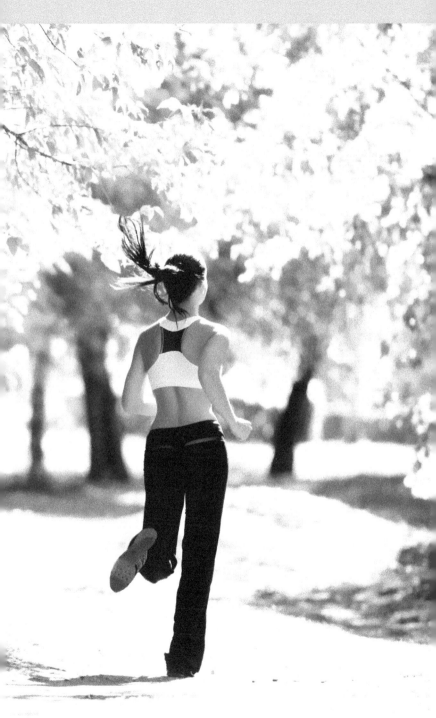

food diary, and a fun program to get you moving. This program is designed to invigorate and energize!

The 49-Day Rejuvenating Program— Wellness Comes Naturally

For a healthier you in just 49 days! Discover how busy people like you can lead healthier, happier lives in just seven weeks or less. If you suffer from frequent infections or viruses, lack of energy, lethargy, depression, chronic fatigue, food addictions or intolerances, or battle with conditions that make you tired and unwell, then this program is for you.

The different phases of the program will take you gently through a bowel and parasite cleanse, digestive rebalancing and a liver cleanse. Your digestive health will be under control, you will be cleansed and feel clearer, lighter and absolutely fantastic.

The suggested menu is packed with superfoods to satisfy and nourish the whole family. This is a fantastic way to learn about real health. This program is not about diets and deprivation—rather, it's an education on the abundance that nature offers and the reasons why you get sick. It comes with over 200 recipes to dazzle your taste buds.

This online program comes with eight handbooks, recipe book, wellness diary, audios and a stack of videos to make the whole learning process more fun. It includes eight weeks of online classroom support with wellness consultants—you don't have to do it alone, we will be there with you every step of the way. It's a great way to take control of your health and stop living the hard way.

Moving Beyond Stress— Home Study Program

Up to 90 percent of chronic disease has stress as the underlying cause. This is a breakthrough way to let go of stress, regardless of financial worries, frustrating colleagues, customers or family dramas. Get to the real core of stress and take control.

The program offers a unique perspective of the inner self—you won't find my "Grace Method" anywhere else. It includes eight online classrooms, along with activities and visualizations, leading you gently to a place of calm, clarity and the feeling of absolute freedom. You will never see yourself or your relationships in the same light again.

The Gold—Indulge in the Ultimate Health Program

This covers it all: Wellness Comes Naturally and Moving Beyond Stress, plus more. This truly is the ultimate combination of physical and emotional health to help heal on all levels. It includes 12 weeks of online classroom support. This program is beautifully boxed and includes eight manuals, ten audio CDs and three DVDs.

As you understand the body-mind connection you can really take control not only of your health and addictions, but all your dreams and desires. For those ready for nothing less than a complete transformation!

Moving Beyond Stress Membership Site

For those who are time-challenged, the Moving Beyond Stress program is offered via weekly e-classes, including visualizations and audios. It includes monthly Q&A online classroom support and offers all the benefits of the home study pack, yet is spaced at an easy pace with time to consolidate and integrate this incredible life-changing information. Letting go of the past has never been so easy.

Moving Beyond Stress Workshop

A condensed version of the Moving Beyond Stress home study program is offered as a two-and-a-half-day workshop. It is packed with activities, visualizations and lots of fun—getting to know the real you has never been so interesting and rewarding.

Practitioner training

A 12-month mentoring program is available by application, for those wishing to teach Moving Beyond Stress using the Grace Method through private consultations or workshops. After a year of working with Susanne and her team, your world and your finances will never be the same.

Health retreats

For those wanting to be thoroughly pampered, cleansed, massaged, supported and educated about themselves like never before.

Contact details

Website: www.letgoandlive.com.au and Sister website: www.movingbeyondstress.com

Email: info@letgoandlive.com.au we are here to help you. You don't have to do it alone.

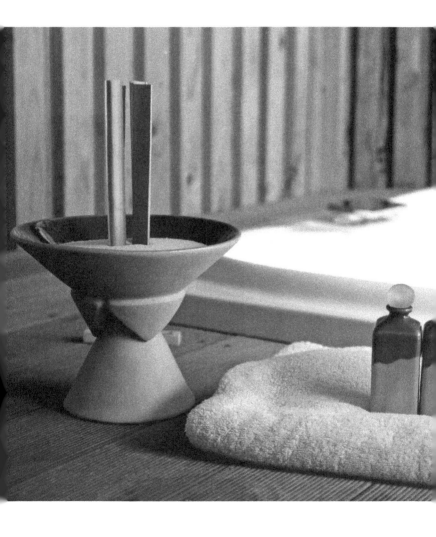

About the author

After 30 years in the health industry as a registered nurse, and years spent struggling with her own health, Susanne Grace became passionate about helping others let go of their pain.

Susanne has a Bachelor of Business, and is a meditation teacher. She is trained in Neuro-Linguistic Programming (NLP), Time-Line Therapy, the MACE Energy Method, Life Coaching and Master Business Coaching, and is certified to deliver Emotional Intelligence training and assessment.

Susanne uses a unique teaching and presentation style to offer information, inspiration and life-changing programs. Combining her own knowledge and experience with that of an expert team of naturopaths, researchers, and natural health practitioners, Susanne has developed Let Go and Live Well and the holistic health programs it offers.

www.ingramcontent.com/pod-product-compliance
Lightning Source LLC
Jackson TN
JSHW071341130125
77033JS00028B/1006

* 9 7 8 1 5 9 1 2 0 3 8 5 8 *